To gain composure,

have the courage to free yourself,

for yoga breaks,

and moments just for you.

© 2007 by GRÄFE UND UNZER VERLAG GMBH, Munich

This 2008 edition published by Metro Books,
by arrangement with GRÄFE UND UNZER VERLAG GMBH, Munich

Layout and cover design:
independent Medien-Design, Munich, Luitgard Schüller
Illustrations: Isabelle Follath, Zurich
Foto on page 126: Studio Arnt Haug, Hamburg
Translation: José Medina
Editor: Kevin White
Production: bookwise Medienproduktion GmbH, Munich

Metro Books
122 Fifth Avenue
New York, NY 10011

ISBN-13: 978-1-4351-0893-6

The exercises described in this book have been carefully researched and tested.
Nevertheless, we cannot guarantee them. We likewise do not assume liability
for any personal, material, or monetary damage.

Printed and bound in China

1 3 5 7 9 10 8 6 4 2

URSULA KARVEN

Yoga on the Go
Exercises and Wisdom for Every Day

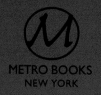

METRO BOOKS
NEW YORK

Contents

Good
Morning!
14

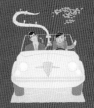

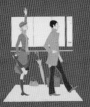

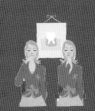

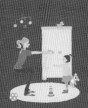

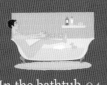

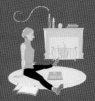

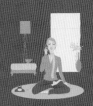

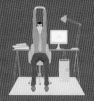

Good
Day to you!
40

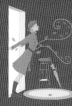

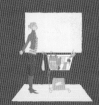

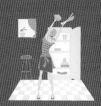

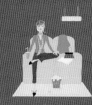

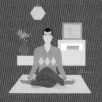

Good
Night!
112

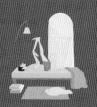

Brief yoga guide

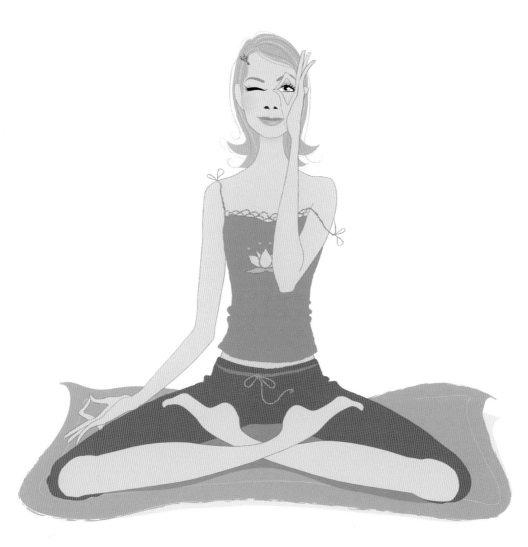

Foreword

While we're all busy trying to manage our lives as efficiently as possible, we often lose sight of the most important thing: ourselves!

Isn't it strange how we have the hardest time letting go when we're under the greatest amount of stress, and how we often don't treat ourselves to a break when we need one the most? Instead, we feel compelled to take care of everything else before we choose to wind down and relax, even when our bodies have been sending clear alarm signals.

We often don't even realize that situations like these actually call for a bit of courage. Indeed, the courage to stop, take a few deep breaths, find our center and then continue working with a fresh sense of self-awareness and revitalized energy.

I would like to remind you that it is up to us to take advantage of the many moments in a day, and not let them pass by unappreciated. We alone determine how we deal with stress. We can include breaks whenever we want, and we can make our energy work for us, instead of against us.

In times of stress or exhaustion, I've often experienced how good it feels to do a simple yoga exercise and spend a moment with myself. I feel better every time. I feel refreshed, concentrated and relaxed. By focusing on my breathing, I have gotten back in touch with my body and am once again connected – online, you could say – with myself.
And that is precisely what I would like to do for you, too!

Namaste.
With all my heart.

"The secret to *freedom* is *courage*« (Pericles)

Namaste

The word "namaste" comes from Sanskrit and means "That which is divine in me bows before that which is divine in you". The accompanying gesture is bringing the palms of the hands together in front of the chest, closing the eyes and lowering the head slightly forward. As a ritual before or after exercises, many yogis first touch the "third eye" – the area on the forehead between the eyebrows – and then the lips before bringing the joined hands to the chest.

This gesture stands for clarity of thought, for the truth of the spoken word, and for the purity of feelings. "Namaste" is a wonderful start to the day.

This is yoga

Yoga is neither a religion nor a dogma. It is a philosophy that has its roots in India. The word "yoga" (like "namaste") comes from Sanskrit and means "union" – in this case, the union of body and soul with the great wholeness of things. Practicing yoga and proper breathing techniques brings everything together, brings you closer to yourself and at the same time reconnects you with your environment. Yoga exercises are called asanas. This book will often use Sanskrit terms with English translations next to them. Many of the exercises are variations on classical yoga asanas, adapted for everyday situations.

>>> Breathing...

Breathing is an essential feature of yoga. It is vital that you concentrate on breathing gently and deeply through your nose. That's just about all there is to it. Imagine exhaling through your open mouth onto a mirror. If you can produce that sound with the same effort – but with your mouth closed – you've already learned "Ujjayi" breathing. This is the yoga breathing technique that best supplies the body with oxygen during exercises.

How to get the most out of the exercises

Before starting an exercise you should collect your thoughts and gather your composure for a moment by focusing attention on yourself and your senses. This quiet moment will help calm you while also increasing your concentration.

Inhale and exhale consciously and deeply through your nose once before starting with the asanas.

>>> Why less is more...

Although most yoga exercises focus on particular parts of the body, their effects are felt all over: muscles are stretched and strengthened, and the blood supply to your organs is stimulated.

It's important to take your time and breathe deeply for each asana in order to experience and absorb the exercise fully. It is better to concentrate fully on a single exercise than to lose yourself in a long routine where your focus may wane. If an exercise or a position causes you pain, be sure to stop immediately.

>>> Why integrate your feelings...

While continuing your breathing, it is important to pause briefly after each exercise. This makes it easier to carry the good feeling into your everyday life. Smile. Then try to take the smile with you. By actively integrating the feeling, you're making the yoga exercises more productive and strengthening their long-term effect.

Letting go of your thoughts

It is important clear your head when doing these exercises. Annoying thoughts will often flash through our minds: a lengthy to-do list with long emails that haven't been sent yet, trouble with the boss or people at work, nervousness about next week's meeting. Forge it all! Don't let these thoughts distract you. Instead, let them flow for a moment. Acknowledge them. Be aware of them. Then let them go. There is no pressure to complete unfinished projects or to find solutions to problems while you are doing the asanas. The object is to breathe and to stretch your body. You can focus on those other things later.

GOOD MORNING!

>>>A few short exercises are a lot better than that nagging guilty feeling.

Hardly anybody has the time to go to the gym every day or attend yoga classes. But exercise should never be neglected, especially when we are under stress. Typically, we come home from work exhausted and would rather lie down on the sofa than do something good for our bodies. How often do we turn off the alarm clock in the morning and stay in bed – despite having made a firm decision to start the day with exercise? Then we feel guilty ... again.

Believe me, it happens to me too, and I'm a huge yoga fan. I often have to wrestle with my weaker inner self when it comes to getting up earlier for my typical 90-minute yoga session. Sometimes it feels as if my arms and legs are full of lead. And in the evening, after a full day of juggling work and kids, I need an hour to relax my overloaded system. Otherwise I fall fast asleep – already a handy excuse for the next morning...

But ever since I released myself from the pressure of doing my training exercises all in one session, my day has become easier and more playful. Of course, I do my full yoga program as often as possible, but I also distribute the exercises over the course of the day if need be. Sometimes I stretch during my tea break. Other times I do a twist exercise in my office chair. Occasionally a hip exercise while watching TV does the trick, or a breathing exercise during film takes. This not only gets rid of that guilty feeling, but it also becomes fun, so I add another exercise, and then another, and one more ... The point is, short breaks are always better than none at all.

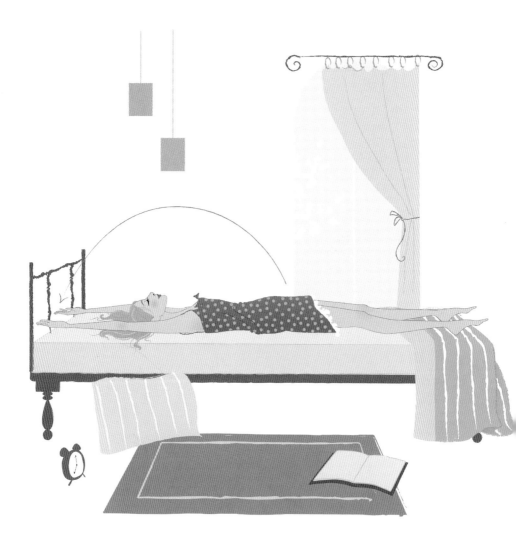

A New Day, a New Start

Urdhva Hastasana variation – Raised Hands variation

>>> How it works...

Lie on your back. While inhaling, bring both arms up and over your head. Stretch as far as you can. Briefly hold your breath. Exhale and bring your extended arms back to your sides. Release.

Repeat at least three times. If you have back problems, bend your knees slightly or place a cushion under your knees.

< < < *The benefits*

Stretches and relieves the spinal column, and thus the spinal disks. Body and mind are invigorated. The conscious, deep breathing increases your powers of concentration.

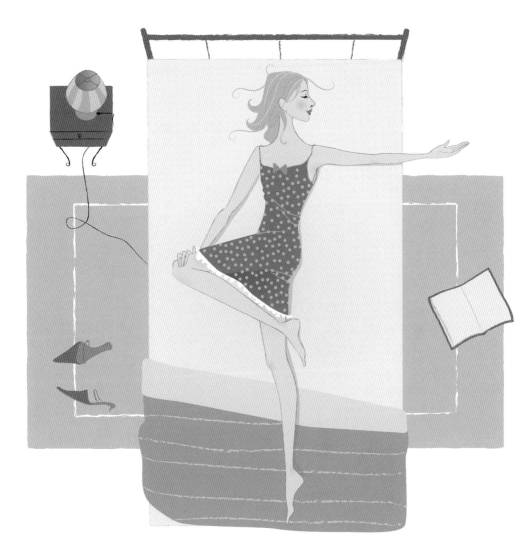

Morning Twist

Jathara Parivartanasana variation – Abdominal Twist variation

>>> How it works...

Lie down and relax on your back. Cup your hands over your left knee and pull it towards your chest. Release your left arm and lay it stretched out to the side. Keep it flat on the mattress. Turn your head to the left. Then, with your right hand on the outside of the left knee, gently pull the left leg over the still outstretched right leg. With each exhaled breath, gently push the knee further down toward the mattress. Keep pushing until you reach the last comfortable position and hold for five to ten deep breaths.

Then slowly relax your body and continue the exercise for the other side.

<<< The benefits

The sides of the body are stretched. The inner organs are stimulated. The body is realigned and straightened.

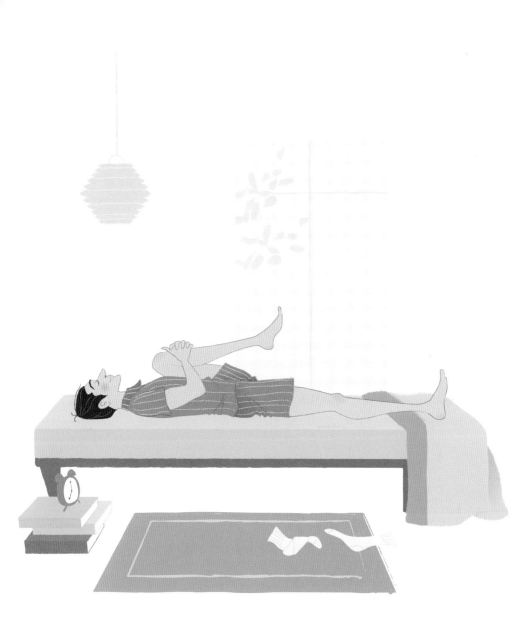

Knee Kiss

Ekapada Pavanamuktasana variation –
Single Knee to Chest variation

>>> How it works...

Lie on your back. Inhale and bend your left knee. Cup both hands over your left knee and gently pull it towards your chest. Leave the right leg relaxed and extended. Inhale and exhale deeply five times in this position. Each time you exhale, try to bring your knee closer to your chest. Lower your leg back to the mattress after the last deep breath.
Repeat the exercise with your right leg.

<<< The benefits

Improves flexibility in the hips. Nicely stretches thigh and buttock muscles.

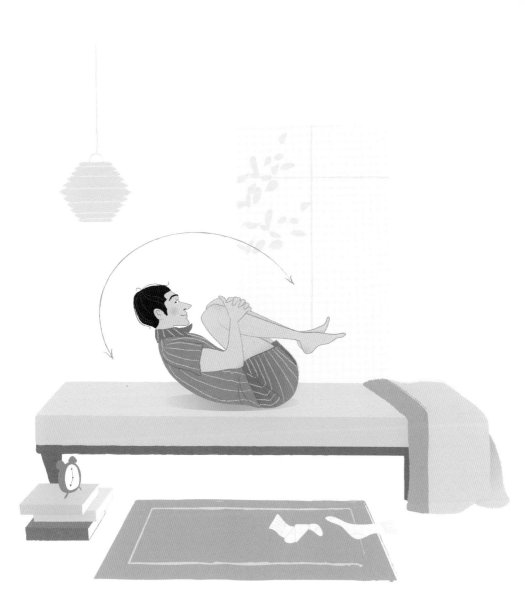

Rocking Up and Down

Dvipada Pavanamuktasana variation –
Double Knee to Chest variation

>>>How it works...

Lie on your back. Inhale and bring your knees up. Wrap your joined hands around both knees and pull them gently towards your chest. Depending on how you feel, you can move your torso in circular or see-saw movements, for example. Then, rock your body up and then back down again as far as you can, like a rocking chair.

Repeat as often as you want, depending on your morning mood.

<<< *The benefits*

Relaxes and stimulates circulation in the entire back. Stretches the shoulder muscles. Firms the abdominal muscles.

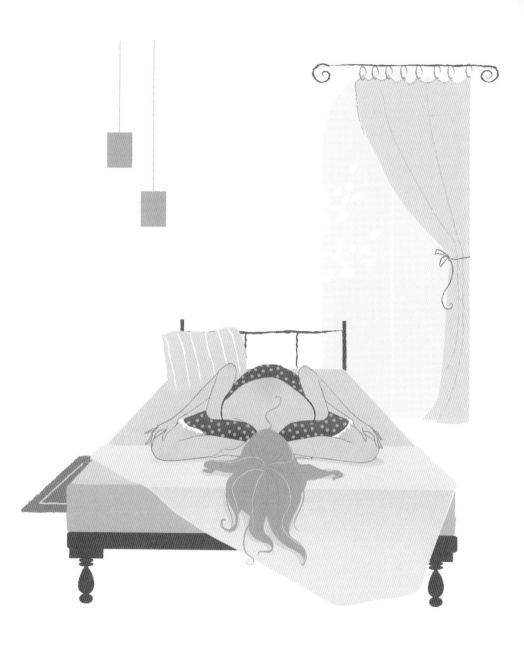

Bowing

Siddhasana variation – The Perfect Pose with Bowing variation

>>> How it works...

Sit cross-legged on the bed with the palms of your hands on your knees.
Inhale deeply and straighten your back. Exhale and bend over forward as far
as you can with your back straight. Then lower your head, round out your
back and shoulders, and try to touch the bed with your forehead. Breathe in
and slowly straighten out your back, one vertebra at a time until your back
is completely erect again.
Repeat the exercise five times.

<<< The benefits
Improves circulation in the head and lower abdominal organs. Stretches
neck muscles. Eases stiffness in the knees and ankles.

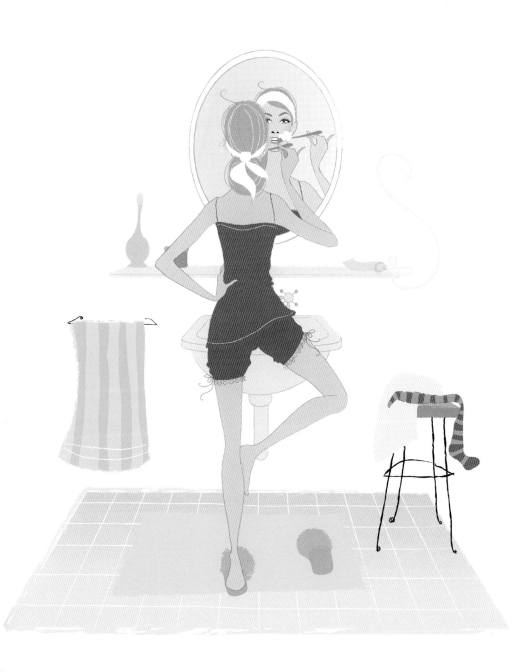

Wide Awake

Vrikshasana variation – Tree variation

>>> How it works

Stand up straight in front of the bathroom mirror. Rest your left hand on the left side of your waist. Focus your eyes on a point directly in front of you. Bend your right leg and rest the sole of your foot on your left knee. Keep your upper body erect and your left leg as straight as possible. Keep your pelvis straight. Brush your teeth with your right hand. Don't forget to smile, and to breathe gently and deeply during the entire exercise.
After about a minute, change sides and rest the left foot on the inside of the right knee. And continue brushing your teeth.

<<< *The benefits*

Improves concentration and equilibrium. Strengthens the leg muscles. Opens the pelvic area. Improves balancing skills.

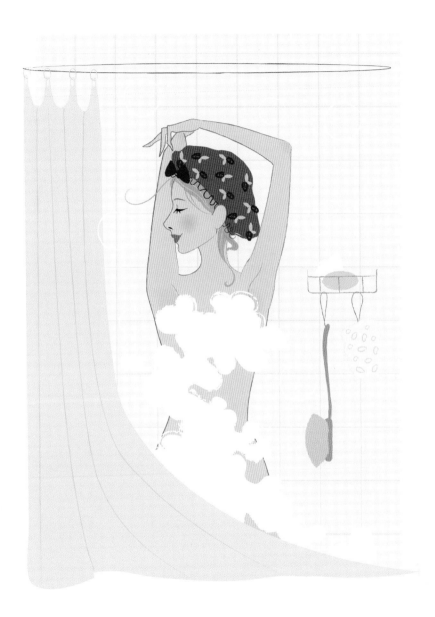

Armpit Inspector

Ardha Gomukhasana variation – Half Cow Face variation

>>> How it works

In the shower, stretch your arms straight upwards. Bend the right arm and bring the palm of your hand down behind your head towards the left shoulder blade. Turn your head to the right and tilt it forward slightly. Grasp your right elbow with your left hand and gently pull to your left side.

Inhale and exhale deeply three times. Switch arms and turn your head to the other side.

<<< The benefits

Stretches the muscles of the arms and shoulders. Relaxes the neck. Activates the shoulder joints.

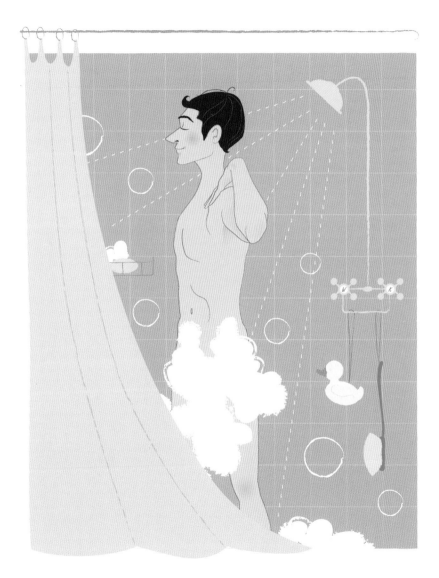

Rain Dance

>>> How it works

With your elbows stretched out to your side, grasp your shoulders with your hands. Your fingers should be in front of your shoulders and your thumbs behind them. Stand with your pelvis straight and your feet at hips' width. Now, just twist your upper body gently from side to side while the water showers down your body. Breathe calmly.

Repeat at least ten times.

<<< *The benefits*

Activates the upper spine. Deepens breathing. Relaxes the neck. Activates the shoulder joints.

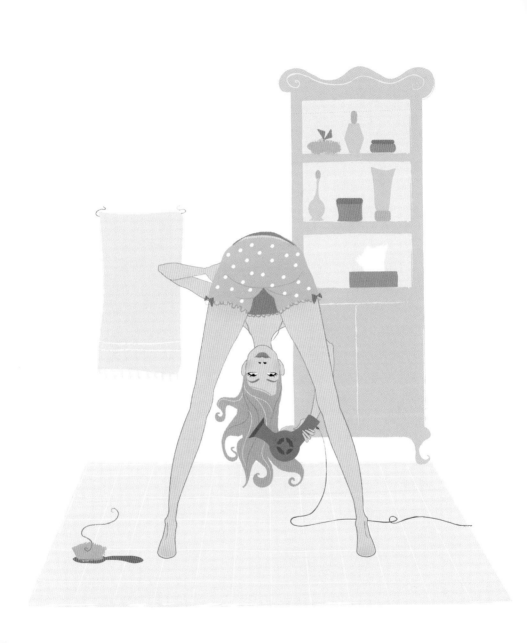

Tailwind

Prasarita Padottanasana variation –
Spread-Legged Forward Bend variation

>>> How it works...

Stand up straight with your hips balanced. Spread your legs wide apart.
Your feet are parallel and pointed forwards. Rest your hands against the
sides of your waist. Inhale and straighten your upper body. Exhale and bend
your upper body out and down to a horizontal position, letting your head
hang loosely. Get the blow dryer and use it as you would typically do. Keep
your legs tense the entire time while bowing forward.
If the stretch in your legs is too intense you can bend your knees a bit.
Inhale and exhale deeply. Each time you exhale, stretch your upper body
forwards a bit more until you have reached the maximum stretch.

<<< The benefits
Improves circulation in the head and upper body. Strengthens thigh, ham-
string and groin muscles. Stimulates digestion.

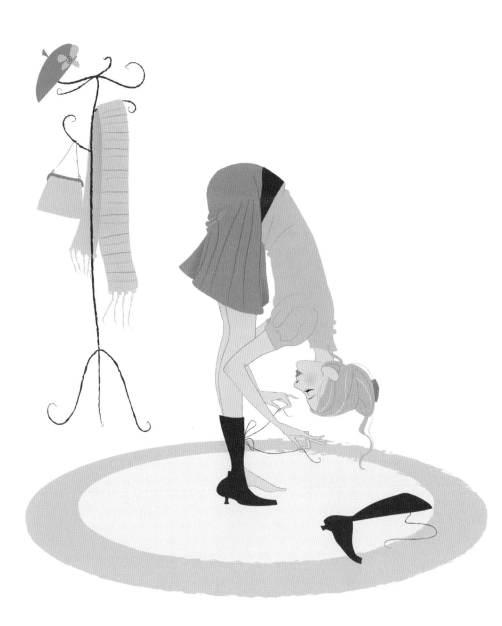

Shoe-Be-Doo

Uttanasana – Forward Bend

>>> How it works...

Stand up straight with your legs slightly apart and your pelvis firm. Inhale, stretch your arms up over your head and bend your knees slightly. Exhale and, with your arms outstretched and your back straight, bend your upper body forward and down. Relax your neck, shoulders and back. Then try to straighten your legs slowly. Inhale and exhale deeply and tie the first shoe. The next time you inhale, keep your knees slightly bent and slowly straighten out your back, one vertebra at a time. Bring your head up last. Repeat the exercise and tie the second shoe.

<<< The benefits

Stretches leg muscles. Strengthens back muscles. Activates the spine. Has a calming effect. Helps combat anger and sadness.

If you are feeling angry or sad, linger over the exercise two minutes with your knees bent. Depending on how you feel, you can fold your arms or let them hang down. Likewise, let your head hang down loosely. Inhale and exhale deeply and calmly.

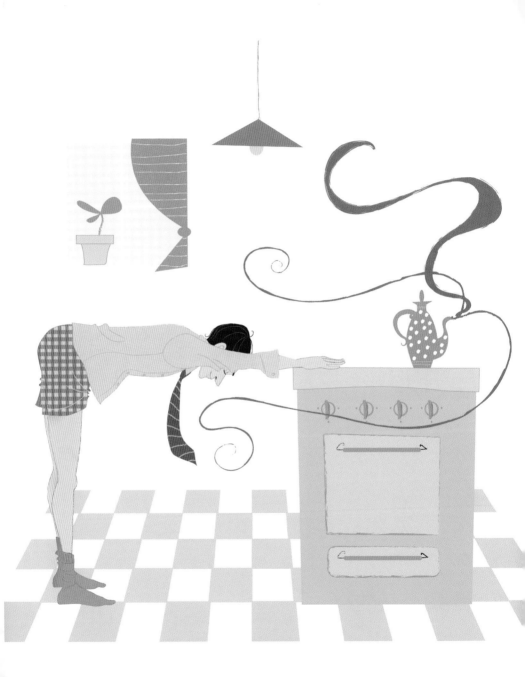

Up and Awake?

Uttanasana variation – Forward Bend variation

>>> How it works...

Stand at least one yard from the kitchen counter with your legs spread as
wide as your hips. Inhale and stretch your arms up over your head. Exhale
and bend your straightened upper body forward. While doing this, flex your
thigh muscles so your kneecaps are being pulled upwards. Rest your palms
on the countertop. Stretch out your back completely. Relax your neck. Your
eyes are facing down. Inhales and exhale deeply.

If the stretch is too intense you can fold your arms, rest your elbows on the
countertop and lay your head on them. Remain in this position for a few
breaths. And enjoy the fragrance of freshly brewed tea or coffee.

<<< The benefits
Stretches back and thigh muscles. Activates the shoulder joints.

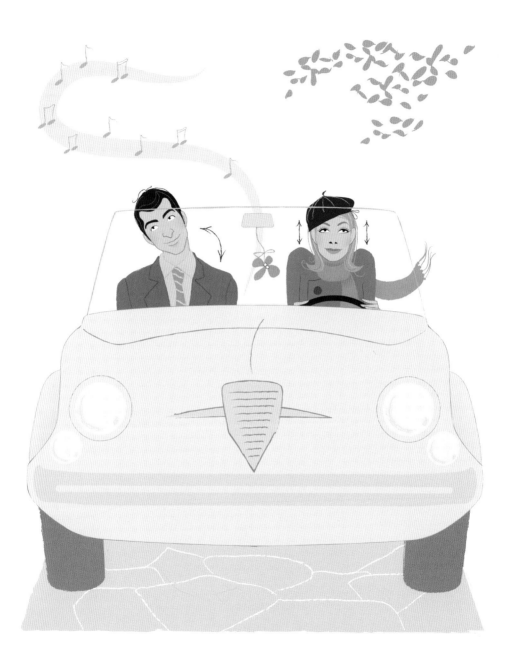

Autogenius Training

>>>How it works...

>>>*Variation I:*

At every red light, straighten your back and upper body. Inhale and pull your shoulders as far up as possible. While exhaling, drop your shoulders agagin. Repeat the movements until the light turns green. You can also rotate your shoulders, three times backwards and three times forwards.

<<< Relaxes the shoulder muscles.

>>>*Variation II:*

Don't let traffic upset you. Straighten your back and upper body. Slowly lower your shoulders. Let your jaw go slack. Tilt your head to the right until you feel tension in your neck muscles. Breathe into this tension three times. Raise your head back to the center and then do the same to the left.

<<< Stretches the shoulder and neck muscles. Relaxes the jaw.

GOOD DAY TO YOU!

>>> The yogis always used to say:
"Breathe slowly, you'll live longer."

"Pranayama" is a Sanskrit term meaning "vital energy". More precisely, it means "the bringing together of body and soul through breathing". Every day we are confronted with challenges and changes, and often we are under tremendous pressure. We should be aware that the more conscious we are of our breathing, the more relaxed and healthy we live. We typically inhale and exhale 18 times per minute. That's 1,080 breaths per hour and 25,920 breaths per day. The yogis of old believed that 21,600 breaths a day would give a person 100 years of life. Everything that speeds up breathing – stress, anxiety, anger – shortens life. So, if you feel you're getting too wound up during the day, take a break, breathe slowly for a minute and, if at all possible, squeeze in a yoga exercise. It is not just the well-being of your mind, but also of your body, that is of paramount importance. Stretch your arms and legs at least once an hour, so all that sitting doesn't get to you.

As an actress, I've worked for over twenty years in front of the camera. Sometimes the camera team is ready for action and the first take is just a few seconds – but I'm just not ready. My heart is pounding, my thoughts are racing and my concentration is gone.

Only over the past few years have I been able to muster up the courage to ask for a minute of patience in those situations, until I've found the right feeling for a particular scene.

Nowadays, even with sixty people waiting impatiently for me, I manage to take a short break, breathe calmly and deeply, and perhaps even go outside for a moment so that I can jump back into the scene. I'm then able to work more efficiently and with much greater concentration, without the actual filming time being any longer for it.

Try it some time in your own work . . . it helps!

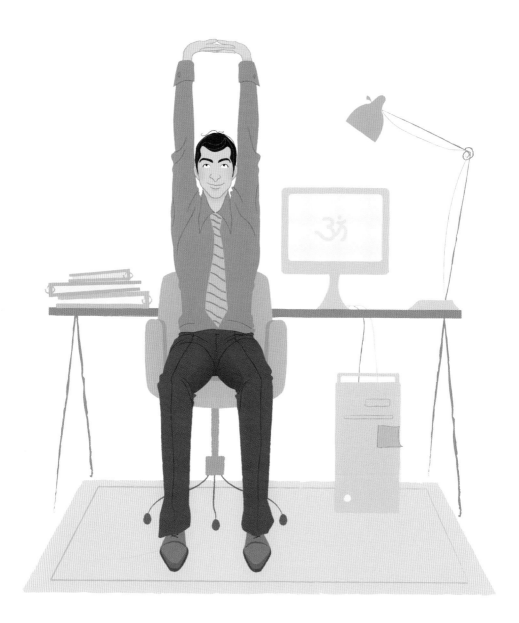

Take Off Like a Rocket

Parvatasana variation – Mountain variation

>>> How it works...

Sit either on your office chair or stand up keeping your your legs at shoulder width. Bring the palms of your hands to your chest. Inhale and slowly stretch your arms upwards until they touch the sides of your head. Exhale and join your hands, intertwining the fingers. Inhale again and stretch your hands upwards, palms facing up. Stretch your arms upwards as far as you can. Then gently exhale and inhale through your nose until the computer is booted up.

<<< The benefits
Stretches shoulder and arm muscles. Lifts and stretches the diaphragm.

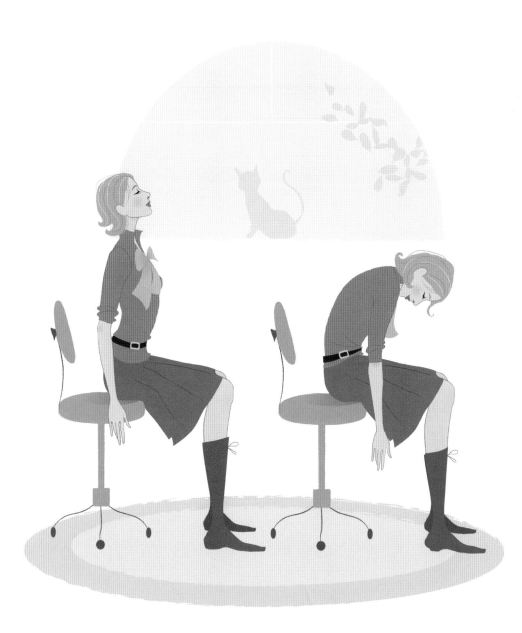

Hot Cat

Cakravakasana variation – Cat variation

>>>How it works...

Move to the front edge of your chair with your legs at shoulder width. Keep
your knees over your heels. Let your arms hang down to your sides. Inhale,
roll your shoulders back, lift your chin up and draw in your lower back.
Exhale and arch your back like a cat, rotate your shoulders forwards, lower
your head, and pull in your belly. The next time you inhale, lift your chest
once more, straighten your spine, raise your chin and look at the ceiling.
Repeat the exercise at least five times.

<<< The benefits
Activates the spinal column. Opens up the chest. Loosens the shoulders.
Deepens breathing.

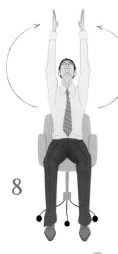

8

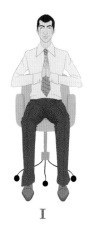

I

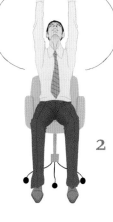

2

Sun
Worshiper

Surya Namaskar variation –
Sun Salutation variation

7

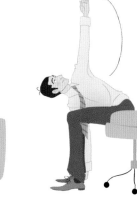

3

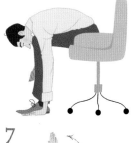

6

5

4

>>> How it works...

Sit on the front edge of your chair. Spread your legs to hip width. Your
knees are over your heels. Fold your hands in a prayer position. **1** Inhale
and exhale deeply through your nose twice. On the third inhale, raise your
hands in a wide circle over your head and look up. **2** While exhaling, keep
your upper body straight and bend forward and down, placing your palms
on the floor next to the outside of your feet. **3** Inhale and raise your left arm
in a semi-circle towards the ceiling. Look up towards your hand. **4** While
exhaling, bring the hand back down to the floor and put it back next to your
left foot. **5** On the next inhale, raise your right arm in a semi-circle towards
the ceiling and look up towards your hand. **6** Exhale and bring your hand
back down to the floor next to your right foot. **7** On the next inhale, raise
your arms in a wide arc up over your head until the palms of the hands
touch. **8** While exhaling, bring the hands down in front of you back to your
chest.

Important: Always keep your back straight and stretched out.

<<< The benefits

Strengthens the muscles of the back and shoulders. Activates the spinal
column. Stretches the chest. Stimulates the digestive tract. Gives you more
energy.

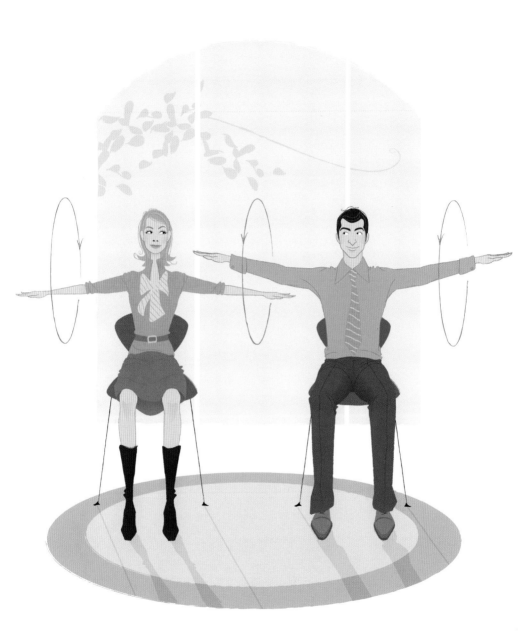

Swingers Club

>>> How it works...

Sit up straight in your office chair. Spread your legs to hip width with your knees directly over your heels. Inhale, raise your arms to your sides and stretch them out as far as you can. Inhale and exhale deeply through your nose while rotating your arms backwards. Begin with small circles, then increase the size steadily. Rotate for at least half a minute. Then change direction.

<<< *The benefits*

Strengthens shoulder and arm muscles.

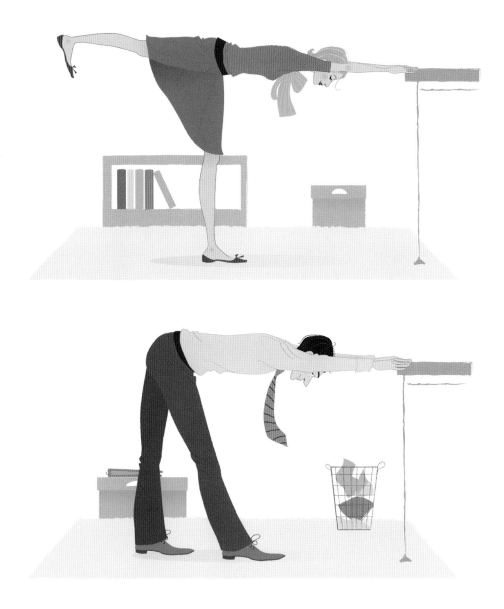

Tae-Kwon-Desk

>>> How it works...

Stand up straight with your legs together. Stay far enough from your desk so you can touch the edge by bending over. Inhale (in variation II the left foot is positioned a small step back) and stretch your arms straight up. Exhale and, keeping your upper body straight, bend forward and rest your fingers on the desk.

>>> *Variation I: Virabhadrasana III variation – Warrior III variation*

On the next inhale, raise your right leg backwards, keeping it extended. Hold for at least five breaths. Switch legs on the next exhale.

<<< Strengthens and stretches the muscles of the buttocks, arms, legs, and feet. Energizes.

>>> *Variation II: Parshvottanasana variation – Side Stretch variation*

Keep your back straight, your neck relaxed and your hips parallel to the table. Hold for five breaths. While exhaling, put your hands on your hips and return to starting position with your back straight. Breathe out and switch legs.

<<< Stretches the muscles of the arms, legs, and hips. Strengthens the abdominal muscles.

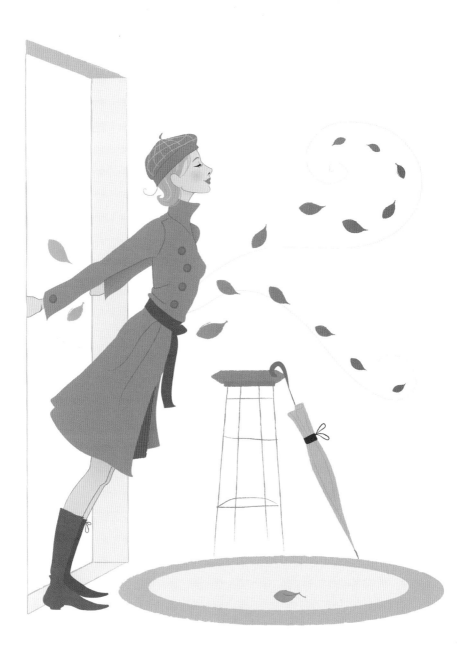

Open, Sesame!

Parshvottanasana variation – Intense Forward Stretch variation

>>> How it works...

Take one step into the room and grasp the door frame firmly to the left and right with your hands. Keep your feet together. Inhale deeply. While exhaling, bring your body forward as far as you can, so that your arms are extended. Then inhale and exhale deeply through your nose while moving your hands slowly up the door frame.

If possible, step back into the door frame and inhale and exhale deeply five times. Then take a step forward again. Relax.

<<< The benefits

Strengthens the muscles of the shoulder blades. Stretches chest muscles. Expands the chest area. Helps combat feelings of fear and anxiety.

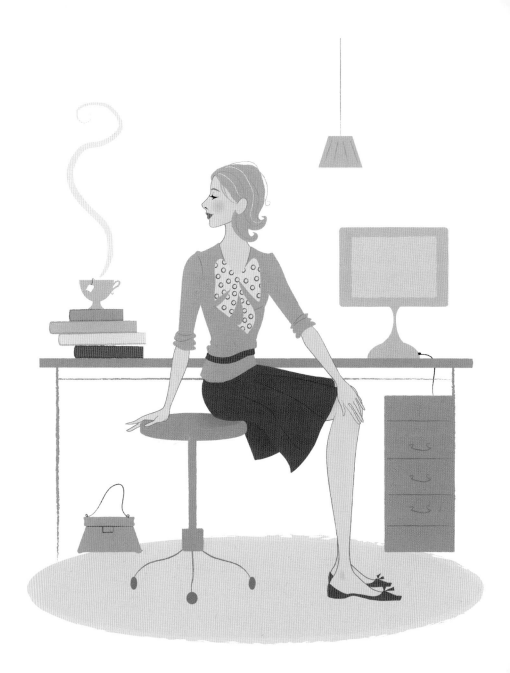

Twisted

Bharadvajasana variation – Swivel Chair variation

>>> How it works...

Sit on the front edge of your chair. Keep your legs together. Put your left palm on the outside of your right knee, keeping your arm straight. Put your right hand on the back of the chair for support with your fingers pointing to the rear. Inhale and stretch your back straight up. Exhale and gently twist your upper body and head to the right. Every time you inhale, stretch slightly upwards, and each time you exhale, twist a bit further to the right. Keep your shoulders relaxed. Inhale and exhale deeply through your nose three times.

Then slowly turn back to the center and do the exercise in the opposite direction.

<<< The benefits

Activates the spinal column. Stretches back muscles, which releases tension. Stimulates the digestive tract. Improves circulation in the organs.

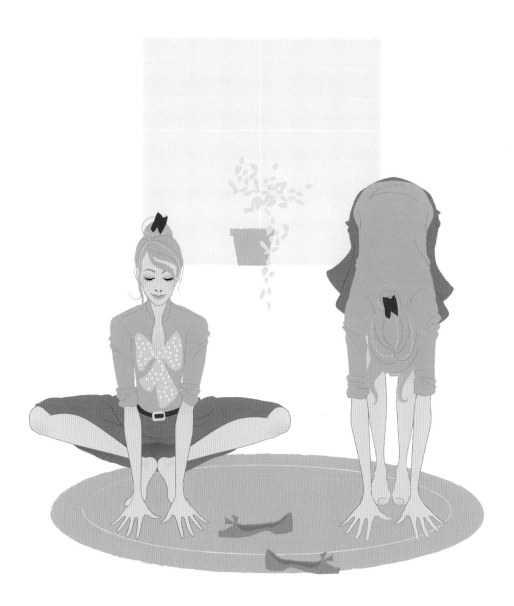

Frog Prince

Mandukasana variation – Frog variation

>>> How it works...

Stand up straight with your legs slightly apart. Squat all the way down with your knees pointing out to your sides and put your palms on the floor directly in front of your feet to support yourself. Balance on the balls of your feet, heels off the floor touching each other. Look down. Inhale deeply. While exhaling, keep your palms and the soles of your feet flat on the floor and raise your buttocks as high as you can. While inhaling, return to the squat position.

Repeat the exercise at least ten times. Keep in mind: Exhale and stretch, inhale and squat back down.

<<< *The benefits*

Promotes flexibility in the hip and pelvic areas. Stretches the muscles in the front and back of the legs.

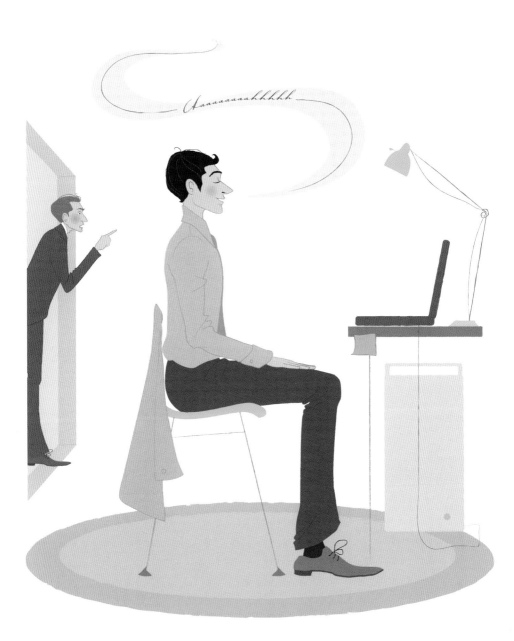

Releasing Pressure

Pranayama variation – Breath and Energy Control variation

>>> How it works...

Sit up straight on your chair with your legs slightly apart and your hands resting loosely on your thighs. Inhale as deeply and intensely as possible through your nose and hold your breath. Inhale again deeply until you get the feeling that your chest is completely filled with air. Keep holding your breath. Then exhale with a loud sigh.
Repeat the exercise three times.

<<< The benefits
Supplies the brain with oxygen. Lifts your mood.

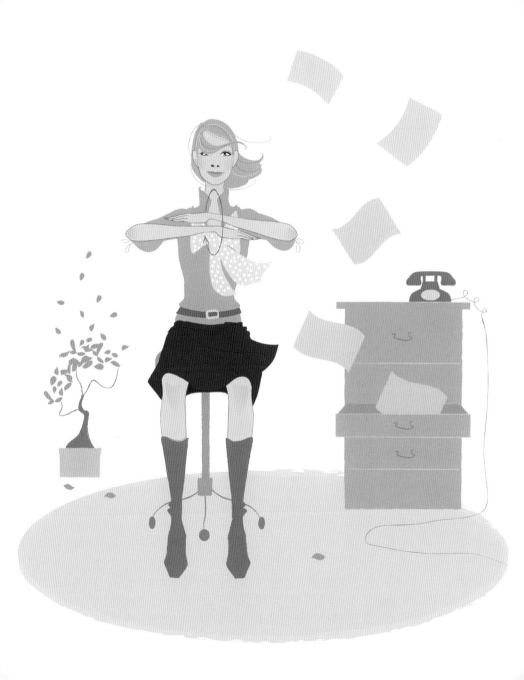

A Fresh Breeze

>>> How it works...

Sit on the front edge of your chair. Your back is straight. Your legs are at least at hip width. Your knees are directly over your heels. Raise your arms in front of you to shoulder level and bend them at roughly a 90-degree angle. Inhale and exhale deeply through your nose while rotating your forearms around each other for about half a minute. Enjoy the fresh air that is fanned from your hands to your face. Make sure that your shoulders are relaxed and pressed down.

<<< *The benefits*

Strengthens the muscles of the chest and arms. Activates the abdominal muscles.

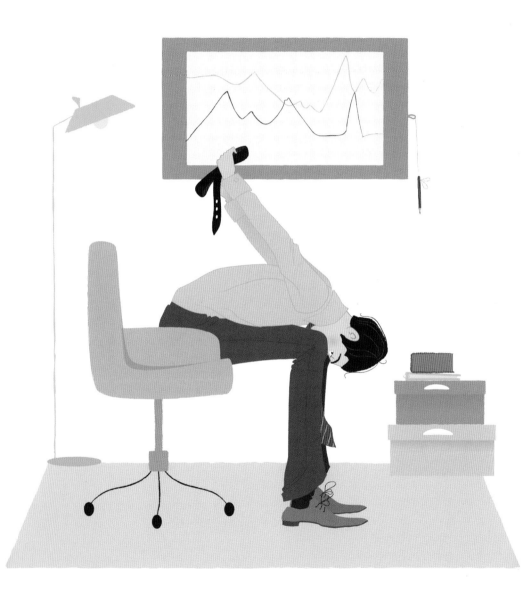

Head Over Heels

Prasarita Padottanasana III variation – Spread-Legged Forward Bend variation

>>> How it works...

Sit on the front edge of the chair. Your legs are open at hip width and your knees are directly over your heels. Hold your hands behind your back. Inhale, straighten your back, and look up towards the ceiling. Exhale and bend forward with your back straight, stretching your arms upwards as far as they can go. Relax your neck. If keeping your hands together is too difficult, you can use a belt.

<<< The benefits

Stretches and relaxes the chest and shoulder muscles. Improves circulation in the head, neck, and shoulders. Increases energy intake.

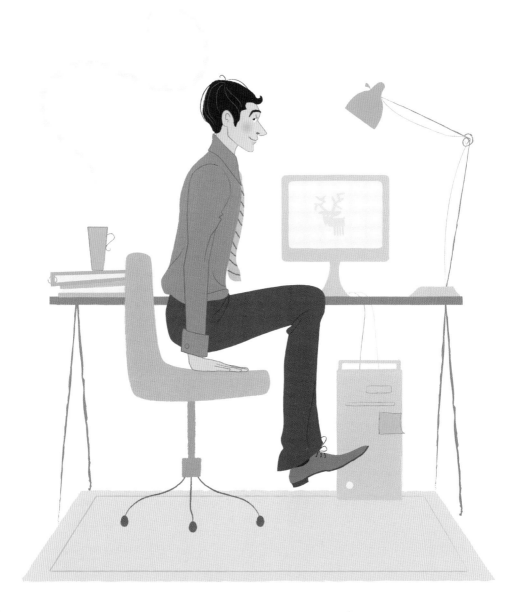

Sitting Pretty

Tolasana variation – Scale variation

>>> How it works...

Sit up straight on your chair with your legs slightly apart. Rest your hands
at your sides. Relax your shoulders. Inhale deeply. While exhaling, tense up
your pelvic floor and arm muscles, and use the combined strength to lift
your buttocks off the seat. Your feet are not touching the floor. Try to hold
the position for three to five breaths. Then lower yourself. Repeat three
times.

<<< The benefits
Strengthens the wrist, hand and arm muscles, abdominal and pelvic
muscles, and the sphincter. Gives you a surge of energy.

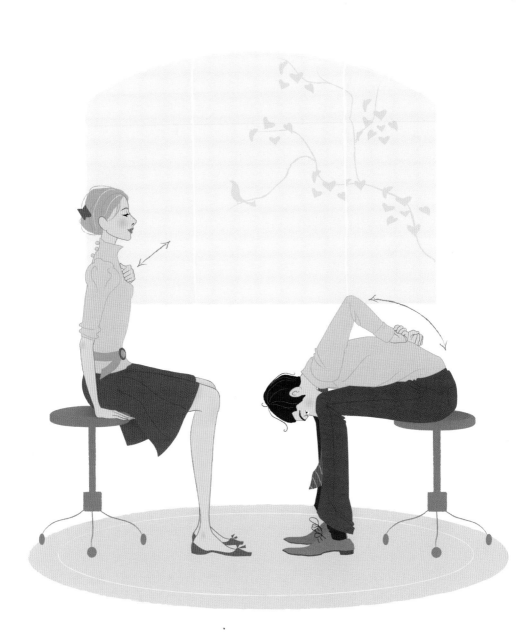

Knockdown

>>> How it works...

>>> *Variation I:*

Sit on your chair with your back straight and your legs slightly apart. Using the palm side of your fist, knock on your breastbone 100 times.

<<< Activates the immune system by stimulating the thyroid gland. Boosts the body's defences and overall well-being.

>>> *Variation II:*

Sit on your chair with your back straight and your legs slightly apart. Bend forward and rest your upper body on your thighs. Let your head hang loosely. Bring your arms behind your back, make fists, and knock gently on your lower back with the backside of your fist, slowly moving up and down your spine for at least one minute. Inhale and exhale deeply through your nose. Slowly sit back up.

<<< Activates the renal cortices, thus improving hormone circulation and resistance to stress.

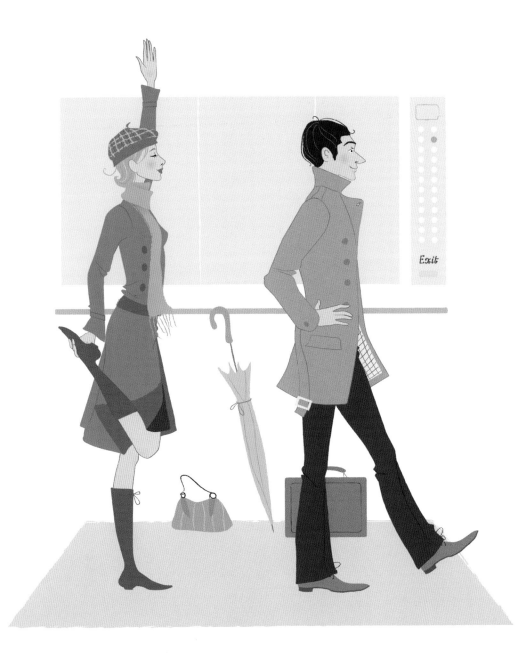

Reach for the Stars

>>> How it works...

Stand up with your back straight, your legs at hip width, and your pelvis flexed.

>>> *Variation I: Natarajasana variation – King Dancer variation*

Fix your gaze on some point in the elevator. Shift your weight to your left leg and stiffen that leg. Bend your right leg back and grasp your right foot with your right hand. Inhale, stretch your left arm all the way up, and balance yourself. Inhale and exhale deeply through your nose five times, then switch legs.

<<< Stretches the muscles of the legs and shoulders. Promotes equilibrium.

>>> *Variation II: Utthita Hasta Padangushthasana – Hand to Foot Extension*

Inhale with your hands resting on your waist. Then exhale, stretch your left leg and raise it slightly. Flex your foot. Focus your eyes on a stationary point and balance yourself. Inhale and exhale deeply through your nose. After five breaths, change legs.

<<< Strengthens leg muscles. Promotes stability.

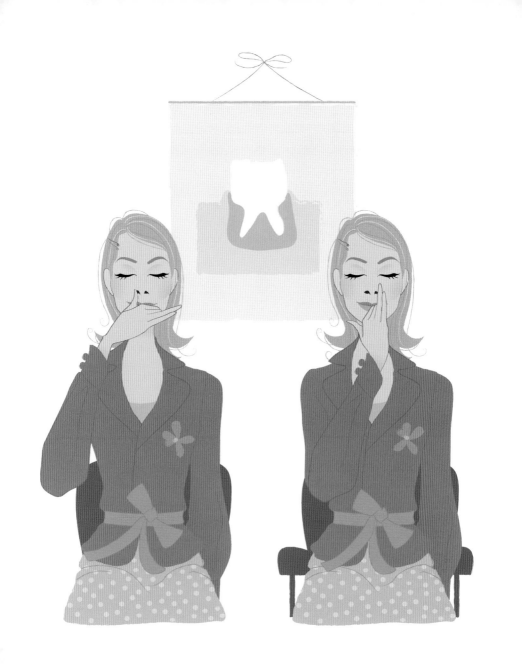

On a Secret Mission

Nadi Sodhana – Alternate Nostril Breathing

>>> How it works...

Sit upright with your legs slightly apart. Keep your back and neck tense.
Close your right nostril with the thumb of your right hand. Your index and
middle fingers are slightly bent, and your ring and little fingers remain
straight. Inhale deeply through your left nostril. Just before exhaling, hold
your ring finger to your left nostril and breathe out from the right nostril.
Then inhale on the right side and exhale on the left side, and repeat . . .
Each time you inhale and exhale, count to at least four. With practice, each
breath can last as long as eight to twelve seconds. The longer and more
even the breath is, the stronger the calming effect becomes. The maximum
effect comes when your exhale time is twice as long as your inhale time
(count the seconds!).
Repeat until any agitation is gone...or until your name is called in the
waiting room.

<<< The benefits
Promotes steady breathing. Helps combat stress and feelings of panic.

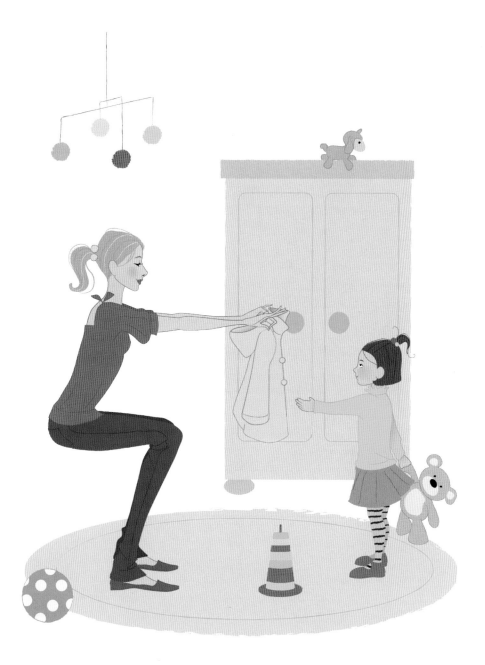

Crouch Down

Utkatasana variation – Sitting with Outstretched Arms variation

>>> How it works...

Stand up straight with your legs slightly apart and your pelvis flexed. inhale and stretch your arms forward at shoulder level. While exhaling, bend your knees and lower yourself. If you can do it, go far enough for your thighs to be parallel to the floor. Shift your weight to your heels. Keep your back as straight as possible. In this position take three to five long breaths. On the last exhale, bring yourself back up. Lower your arms.
Repeat the exercise three times.

<<< The benefits
Strengthens leg and foot muscles. Activates abdominal and back muscles.

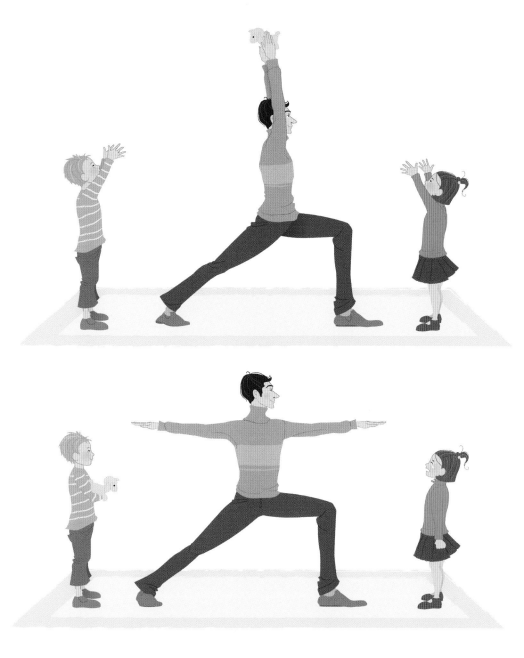

Referee Stretch

Virabhadrasana I and II – First and Second Warrior

>>> How it works...

For the First Warrior: Stand up straight on a NON-SLIPPERY surface and inhale deeply. While exhaling, take a large step forward with your left leg and rotate your right foot inwards to a 45-degree angle. Your heels are lined up and your torso is facing forwards. Inhale and stretch both arms above your head with your shoulders relaxed. Exhale and bend your left knee. Keep your upper body and pelvis straight. Stay facing straight ahead. Hold for at least five breaths before straightening out your legs.

For the Second Warrior: If you want, you can turn the toes of the right foot outwards a bit. Lower your arms to shoulder level, and once again bend the left knee. Your hips are now turned to the side. Hold for five breaths. Inhale, stretch out your left leg and turn the right foot so it faces forward. Turn to the opposite side and repeat both exercises from this position.

<<< Strengthens the ankles as well as the muscles of the knees, legs, shoulders and arms. Invigorates the pelvic and abdominal muscles and the sphincter.

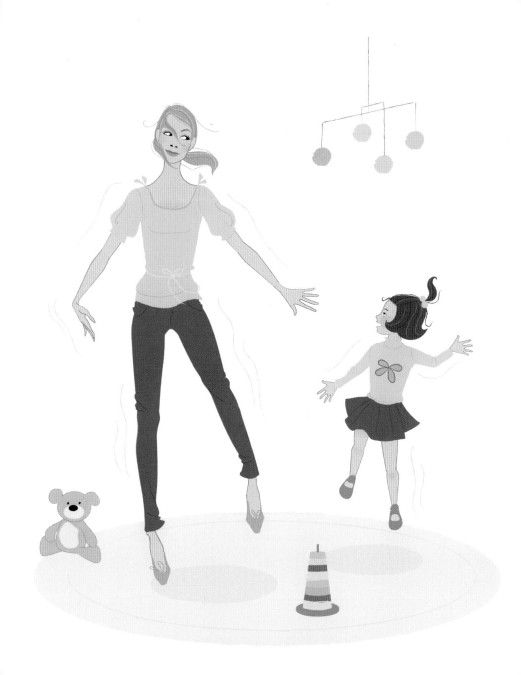

Live Wire

>>> How it works...

Stand up straight and inhale deeply through your nose. Then shake your whole body. Arms, hands, legs, feet, everything. Keep breathing! Shake for as long as it takes to relieve any tension. If you want, you can also yell at the same time. It's even more of a release.

<<< The benefits

Rids the body of tension. Helps combat stress. Lifts your mood.

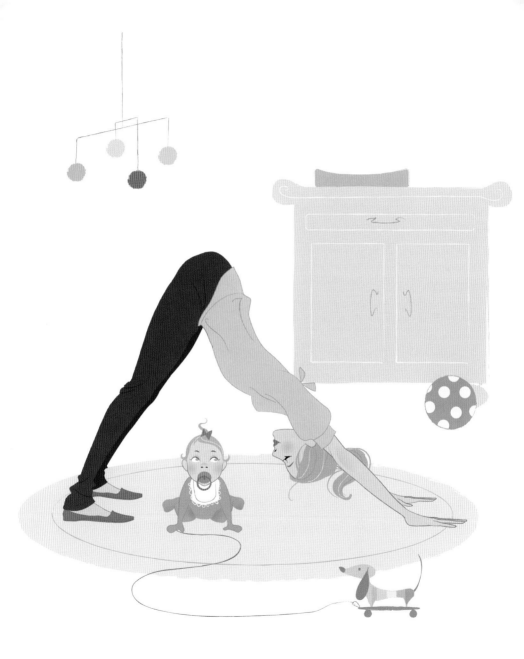

Move, Mama!

Adho Mukha Shvanasana – Downward Facing Dog

>>> How it works...

Get down on all fours with your hands flat on the floor below your shoulders. You can spread your fingers out if you want. Your neck is relaxed. Inhale, get up on your toes and stretch your arms. While exhaling, slowly raise your buttocks and try to extend your legs fully (you may have to move your hands forward a bit).

After some practice, try to stretch your heels slowly towards the floor. Remain in this position for two minutes, breathing quietly and deeply through your nose.

<<< The benefits

Strengthens the joints in the foot and muscles in the legs. Stretches the abdominal muscles. Eases stiffness in the shoulders. Slows down the heart rate and has a calming effect. Invigorates the brain.

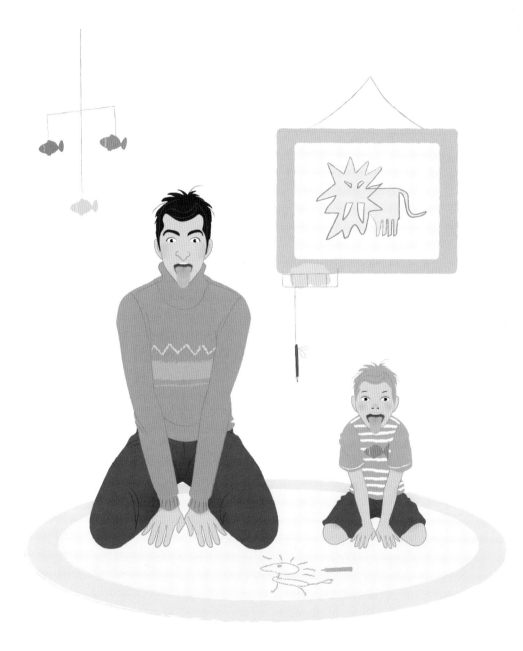

Say Ahhh!

Simhasana – the Lion

>>> How it works...

Kneel down on the floor with your legs slightly apart. Sit on your heels.
Prop your hands on the floor between your legs and straighten your back.
Inhale deeply through your nose, open your mouth and stick your tongue
out as far as possible. Look down at the tip of your nose. Now breathe in
and out through your mouth.
Do the exercise for about half a minute.

<<< The benefits
Calms. Reduces anger and dispels aggression.

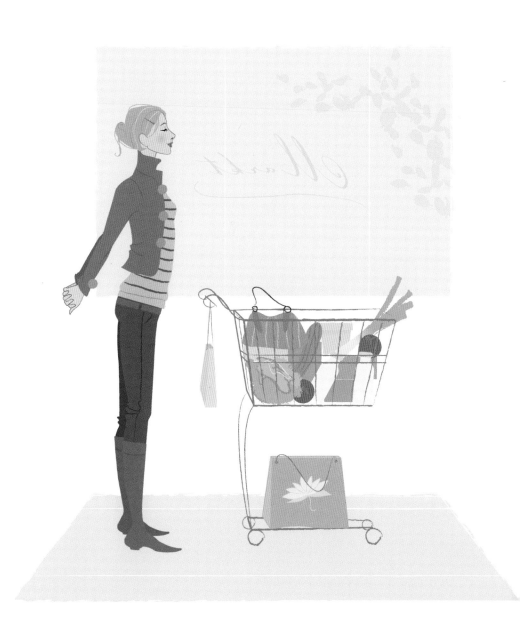

Get It Off Your Chest

>>> How it works...

Stand up straight with your legs slightly apart and your pelvis flexed. Clasp
your hands together behind your back. Inhale deeply through your nose
and straighten your back. While exhaling, stretch your arms upwards as far
as you can. Inhale gently into the stretch.
And don't forget to smile.

<<< *The benefits*

Stretches the muscles of the neck and shoulders. Adjusts and opens the
chest area.

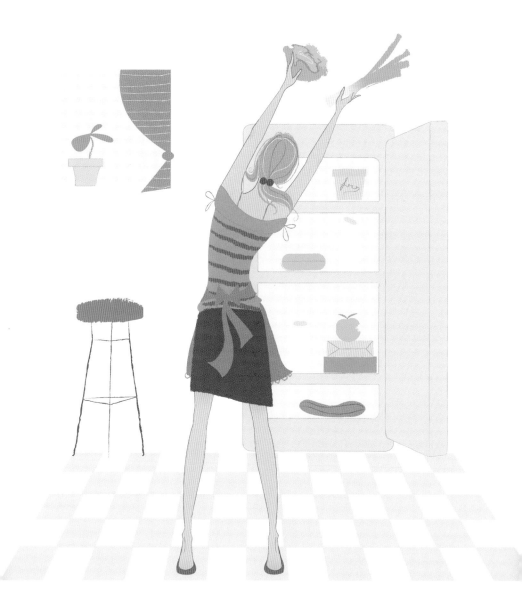

Salad or Vegetables?

Nitambasana variation – Side Stretch variation

>>> How it works...

Stand up straight with your legs at hip width and your pelvis straight.
Breathe in and stretch your arms above your head with the palms of your
hands facing each other. While exhaling, stretch your upper body as far to
the right as you can. You'll feel the stretch along the entire left side of your
body. Hold the position for five breaths. On the next inhale, go back to the
center. On the next exhale, stretch your upper body to the left.
Hold for another five breaths, during which you can calmly think about
what to cook for dinner.

<<< The benefits
Stretches and strengthens lateral elements and muscles of the body.
Stretches the pelvic area. Tightens the belly.

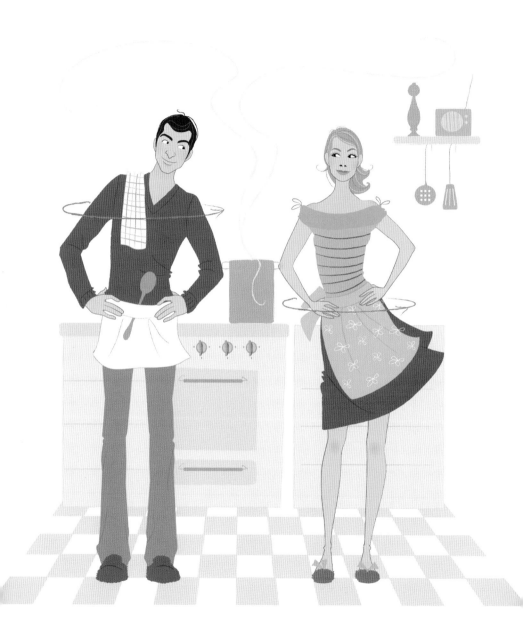

Stovetop Boogie

>>> How it works...

Stand up straight with your legs at hip width and your pelvis flexed. Put your hands on your hips.

>>> *Variation I:*

Inhale deeply. While exhaling, move your torso making small circles, first to the left, and then to the right. Keep your pelvis stable. Keep rotating until the pasta is "al dente".

<<< Activates the entire torso.

>>> *Variation II:*

Inhaling and exhaling deeply, slowly make circles with your hips. First rotate to the left, and then to the right. Now and then, stir the pot. It's also great to rock to the rhythm of music.

<<< Mobilizes the lower back. Strengthens the abdominal muscles.

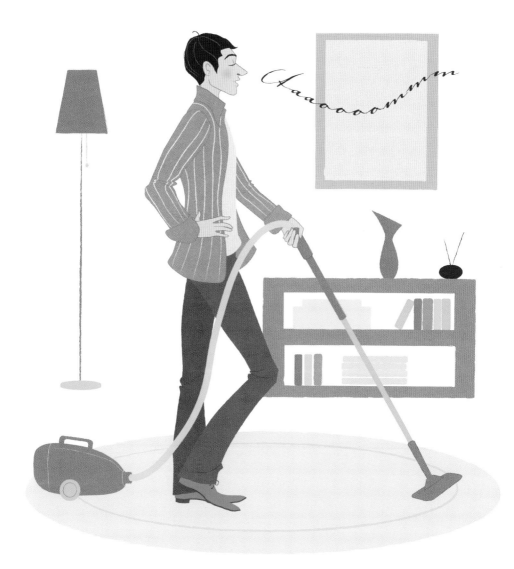

Vacuum Meditation

Chanting mantras

>>> How it works...

The vacuum cleaner is on and nobody can hear you. That's a good thing, since you'll be making plenty of noise as you relax. Here's how you do it: Inhale deeply, open your mouth slightly, and in one long exhaling breath let out a deep, loud AAAHHH. This turns into an OOOHHH. Then slowly close your mouth and let the sound die away as an MMMMMM. You should feel a light vibration in your chest and head while doing this.

<<< The benefits

Calms and relaxes. Deepens breathing. Slows down the brainwaves. Combats stress.

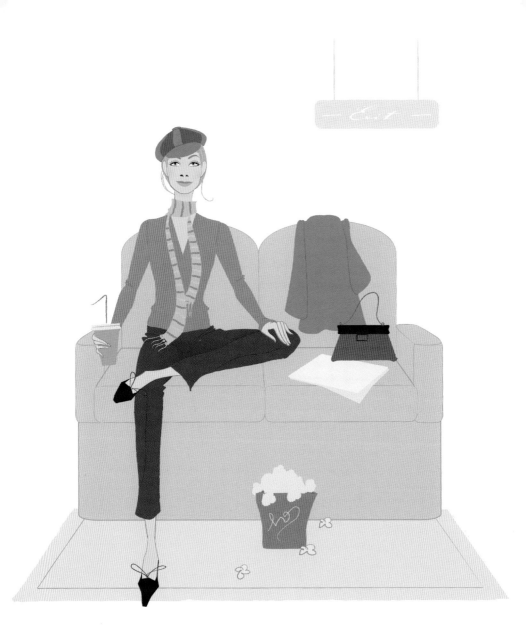

Great Cinema

Padmasana – Preliminary Lotus

>>> How it works...

While at the movies, sit up straight and rest your left foot on your right knee. With your left hand, press down gently on your left knee while inhaling and exhaling deeply. Relax and immerse yourself in the film. Nobody will notice that you're doing yoga.

After a while, switch legs.

<<< *The benefits*

Stretches the inner thigh muscles. Adjusts the pelvis. Opens the hip area. Relieves the lower back.

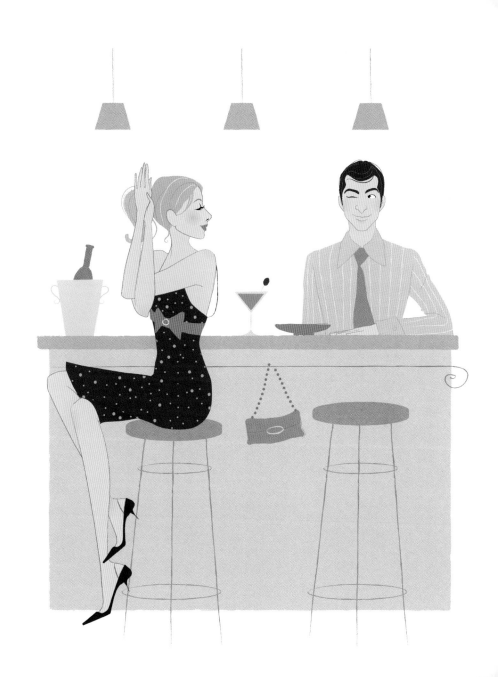

Landing Approach

Garudasana – Eagle variation

>>> How it works...

Sit on a bar stool. Bend your arms and wrap your right arm around your left arm. Lift your elbows up to shoulder level if possible. Now raise your left leg, cross it over your right leg and wrap your foot around your right calf – if you can. Inhale and exhale deeply through your nose. Hold this position for about thirty seconds and focus sweetly on the handsomest man at the bar. Then switch arms and legs, and do the exercise on the other side of your body. Incidentally, the most effective version of this asana is in a standing position, as a balancing exercise.

<<< The benefits
Strengthens the ankles. Stretches and strengthens all the leg muscles. Stretches the shoulder muscles. Activates the spinal column. Strengthens the upper arms.

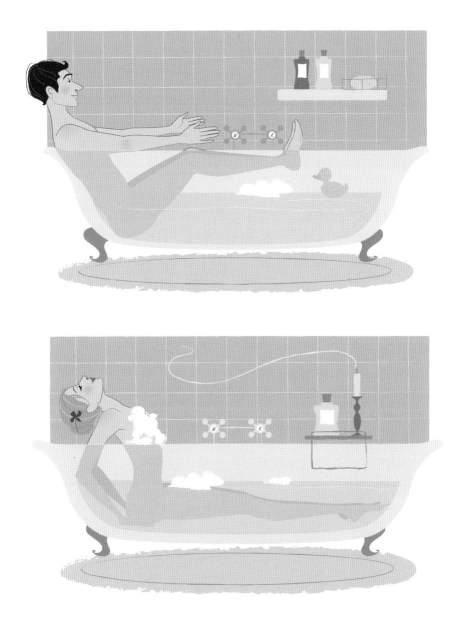

Swimming Champap

>>> How it works...

>>> *Variation I: Navasana variation – Boat variation*
Sit down and lean back at one end of the bathtub. Raise your arms to shoulder level and keep them stiff. The palms of your hands are facing each other. Breathe in deeply through your nose and raise your legs, with your knees slightly bent. Hold for three to five breaths while inhaling and exhaling quietly.
<<< Strengthens the muscles of the abdomen, arms and legs.

>>> *Variation II: Matsyasana variation – Fish variation*
Sit up straight in the bathtub. Put your elbows behind you against the back of the tub and your hands on the bottom of the tub. Inhale deeply. While exhaling, push your shoulder blades back and arch your back. Inhale and slowly stretch your head back. Exhale with a loud sigh with your head still tilted back. Inhale deeply and exhale with a sigh two more times. Then slowly bring your head forward and relax your shoulders.
<<< Stretches the back and chest areas as well as the neck muscles.

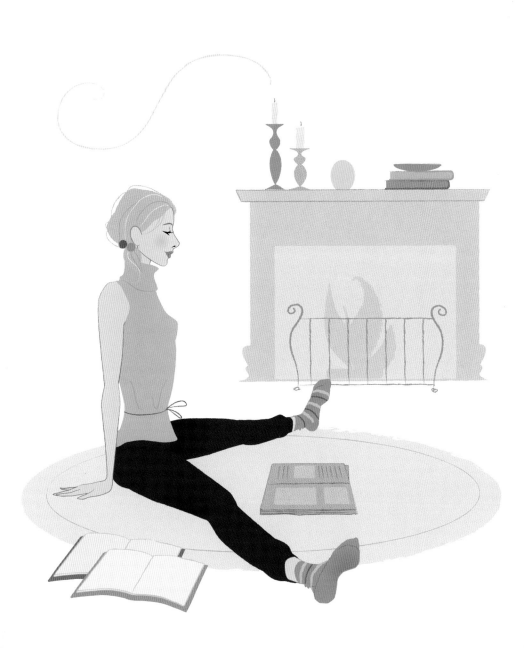

Read and Stretch

Upavishtha Konasana – Seated Angle Stretch

>>> How it works...

Sit down on the floor and spread your legs apart as wide as you can. Flex your feet. Put your hands flat on the floor behind you near your buttocks, with the fingertips pointing back. Straighten out your back.

If you want more stretching, carefully bend forward with your back straight. Keep your neck relaxed. Now quietly read the newspaper.

If you want to stretch even more, bring your hands forward as far as you can and lay them on the floor. See if you can lay your forearms on the floor. (Congratulations!)

<<< The benefits

Stretches and shapes the hips and inner thighs. Improves circulation in the pelvic region. Stretches the lower back. Tightens the belly.

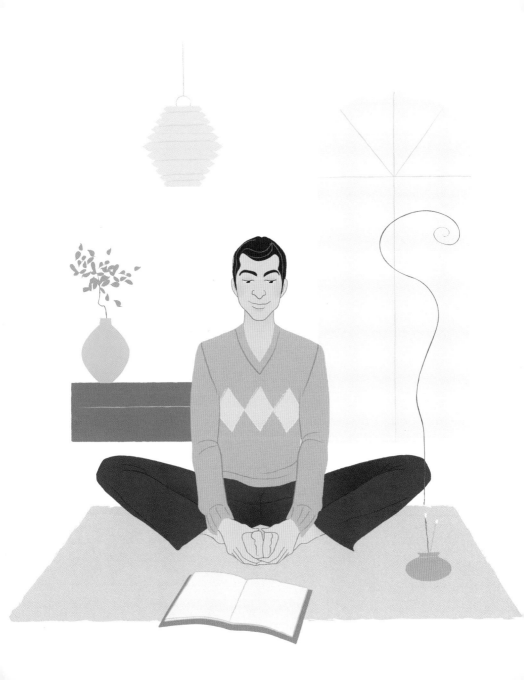

O Sole Mio!

Buddha Konasana variation – Sitting Angle variation

>>> How it works...

Sit on the floor and bend your legs so that the soles of your feet are touching each other. Grasp your feet with your hands and pull them as close to you as you can. Straighten and raise your upper body. If you want more stretching, try to turn your soles up by gently pressing your knees down with your elbows and bending forward as far as possible. Then grab a book and start reading. Inhale and exhale deeply throughout the stretch.
If this is too difficult for you, place a folded blanket or cushion under your buttocks.

<<< The benefits
Stretches the pelvis and back. Opens up the hip region. Improves circulation in the abdominal organs.

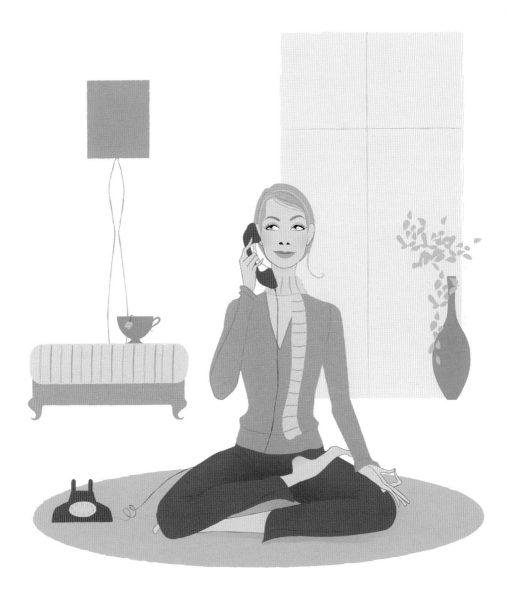

Hot Line

Arda Padmasana – Half Lotus

>>> How it works...

Sit on the floor with your legs stretched out. First bend your right leg and lay your right foot on your left thigh. Your heel should be facing upward, if possible. Then bend your left leg and lay it underneath the right leg. Straighten your upper body and call a friend. Put your free hand on your knee. Touch your thumb to your index finger. The remaining three fingers are spread out. Inhale and exhale slowly and deeply. Switch legs for the next call.

<<< *The benefits*
Relieves stiffness in the knees and ankles. Improves circulation and strength in the lower abdomen organs. Strengthens the spinal column. Relaxes the body while keeping your mind alert.

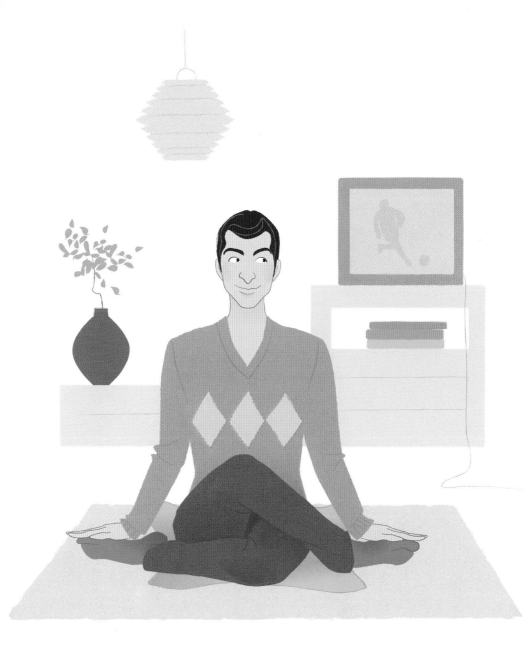

TV Guru

Gomukhasana variation – Cow Face variation

>>> How it works...

Sit on the floor with a cushion under your buttocks and spread your legs.
Bend your right knee and cross your right leg over your left knee so that
your right foot is next to your left hip. Lean a bit to your left and support
yourself on your left hand. Now bend your left leg under you and place your
left foot next to your right hip. Lay the palms of your hands on the soles of
your feet.
Inhale and exhale deeply through your nose, straighten your back, relax
your shoulders and indulge in your favorite TV programme.

<<< The benefits
Stretches the leg and hip muscles. Opens up the hip region. Aligns the back.

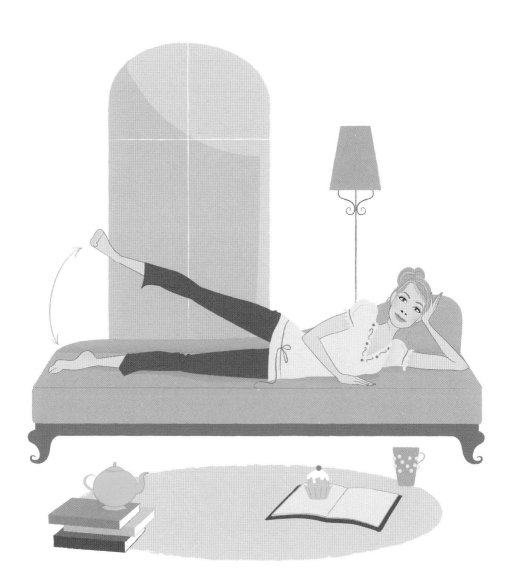

Scissors

Anantasana preliminary pose – Preliminary Side Kick Stretch

>>> How it works...

Lie down on the sofa on your left side and rest your head on your left hand. Place your right hand in front of your upper body. Inhale and exhale deeply. On the next exhale, slowly lift your right leg while counting to five. While exhaling, slowly lower the leg in five steps. Repeat the exercise ten times. Then lie on your right side and do the same with your left leg.

<<< The benefits

Strengthens the leg muscles. Relieves back pain. Strengthens the inner thigh muscles.

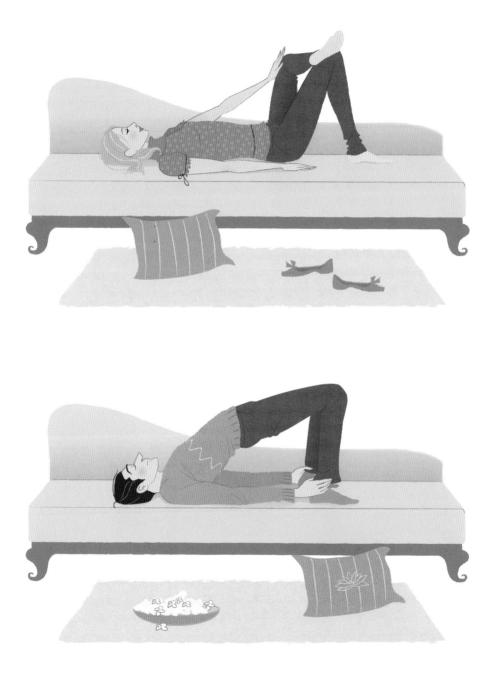

Stretch Break

>>> How it works...

>>> *Variation I: Ardha Padmasana variation – Half Lotus variation*
Lie down on the sofa. Bend your legs upwards. Tense the left foot and rest it
on the right knee. With your left hand press the left knee out. Always
breathe in and out deeply and slowly through your nose. Then switch legs.
<<< Opens the hip area. Stretches the hamstrings. Activates the abdominal
muscles.

>>> *Variation II: Chatur Padasana – Simple Arch*
Lie down on the sofa. Bend your knees upwards. Your feet are apart at hip
width. Bring them close to the buttocks. If you can, grasp the heels with
your hands. Your knees are directly over your heels. Breathe in deeply.
While exhaling, lift first the pelvis and then the entire lower body as high as
you can. The head, neck and shoulders remain relaxed. Hold for at least five
breaths. Then come back down, one vertebra at a time.
Repeat the exercise three times.
<<< Activates the spinal column. Stretches the cervical spine and the loins.

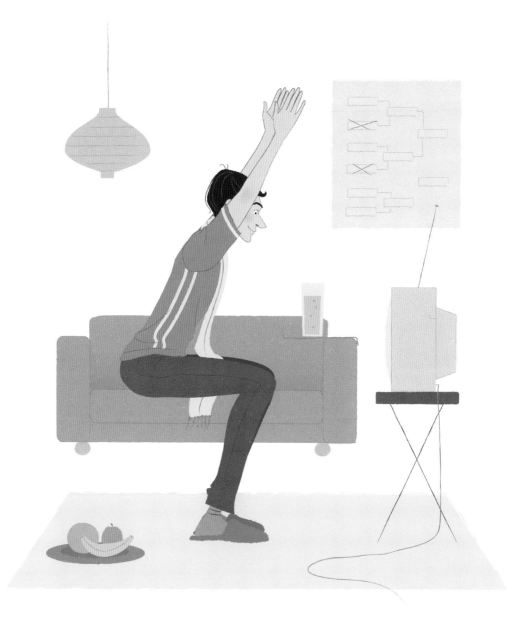

Goal!

Utkatasana variation – Sitting with Upstretched Arms variation

>>> How it works...

First pray, then cheer! Go into a prayer position: legs together, back and pelvis straight, the palms of your hands joined in front of your chest. Inhale and squat down while raising your arms in a broad circular motion. Ideally, you should lower yourself until your thighs are parallel to the floor. Shift your weight onto your heels. Keep your back as straight as possible and lean back in a straight line as far as you can. Remain in this position for three to five breaths. With the next exhaled breath, slowly straighten out your legs. Once you are up, exhale and bring the palms of your hands back in front of your chest.

<<< The benefits

Strengthens the leg and foot muscles. Strengthens the abdominal and back muscles. Improves circulation in the organs. Lifts the diaphragm. Stretches the chest area. Loosens the shoulder muscles.

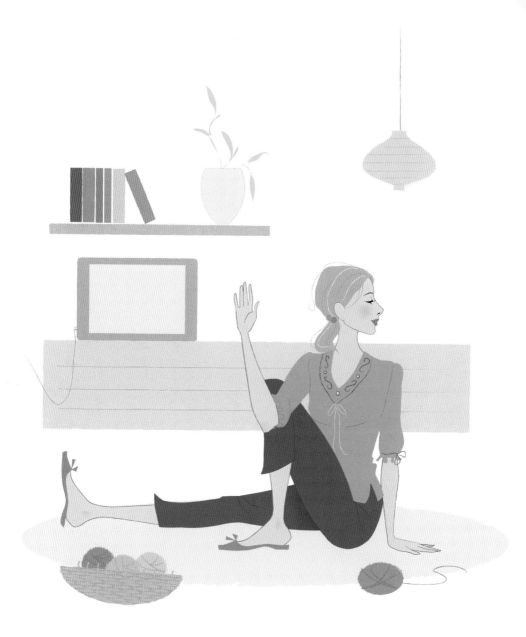

TV Twist

Parivritta Marichyasana – Sitting Rotation with Stretched Leg

>>> How it works...

Sit on the floor with your legs stretched out in front of you and your toes pointing up. Bend your left leg and pull your heel towards you as far as you can. Rest your left hand on the floor just behind your buttocks with your fingers pointing backwards. Your shoulders are relaxed. Now place your right elbow on the outside of your left knee. Inhale and exhale deeply through your nose. While inhaling, straighten your torso. While exhaling, twist your body to the left. Do this three times: inhale and straighten the torso, exhale and twist. Slowly release.
Repeat the exercise on the other side of your body.

<<< *The benefits*
Activates the spinal column and hips. Stretches the muscles in the shoulders, chest and buttocks. Stimulates digestion. Deepens breathing.

GOOD NIGHT!

>>> You can see it all kinds of ways.
Or you can simply think about what you have.

Is the glass half full or half empty? The happiest and wisest people I've
met on my journey through life tend to follow the "half full" theory.
A Tibetan monk once gave me a piece of advice. He told me to give thanks
every evening for everything I have, and not make the mistake of concen-
trating on things or circumstances that I do not have or cannot control. So,
I sat down with him and listed everything I had taken for granted in my
life, from good health and the good fortune to live in a free and democratic
society, to the knowledge that my family has enough to eat and a roof over
its head.

Every time I do this mental exercise I see clearly how thoughtlessly I sometimes deal with the gifts that are bestowed upon me daily. Everything then becomes new to me and I experience humility and the joy of living. Yoga helps me to maintain this feeling. After only a few short exercises (the ones I'm showing you in this book) I can feel how I'm able to appreciate each and every breath, and how conscious breathing calms my soul and gives me inner peace.

One of these evenings, try thinking of all the positive things the day has brought you. You'll notice that it's not a small amount.

And sleep well!

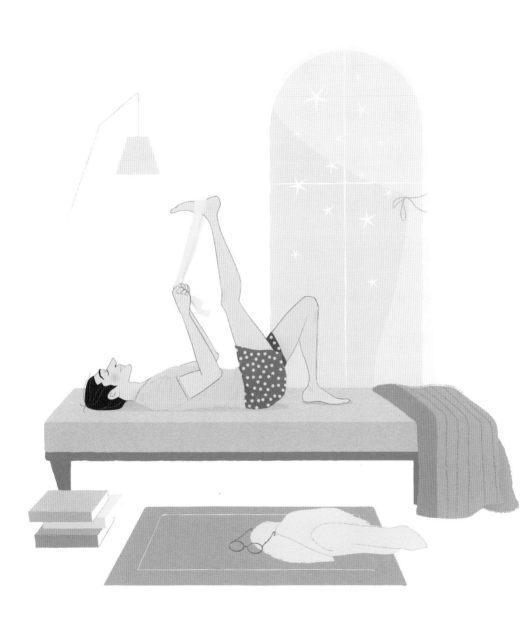

Stretch & Yawn

Supta Padangushthasana variation – Reclining Leg Stretch variation

>>> How it works...

Lie on your back with your knees bent. Sling some sort of belt around your right foot. Inhale and stretch your right leg out and up towards the ceiling. Exhale and use the belt to pull your extended leg slowly towards your chest. When you've reached your limit, breathe into the stretch up to ten times. Then slowly lower the leg back down. Repeat the exercise on the other leg. Important: Make sure your entire back remains flat on the mattress.

<<< The benefits

Stretches the leg muscles. Improves circulation in the legs and hips. Activates the hip joints.

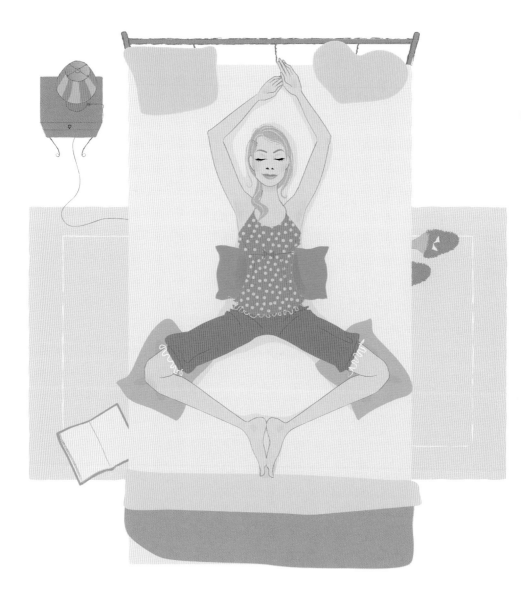

Nocturnal Moth

Supha Buddha Konasana variation – Reclining Angle variation

>>> How it works...

Lie relaxed on the bed. Bend your knees and bring the soles of the feet together. Place a pillow under each knee and another one under your back. Make sure your buttocks are still touching the mattress. Then either stretch your arms out to the side or place them loosely behind your head. Inhale and exhale gently and deeply through your nose. Let go of all your worries.

<<< *The benefits*

Stretches the pelvis and back. Opens the hip area. Improves circulation in the abdominal organs. Relaxes the thigh muscles. Opens up the chest area. Calms you down.

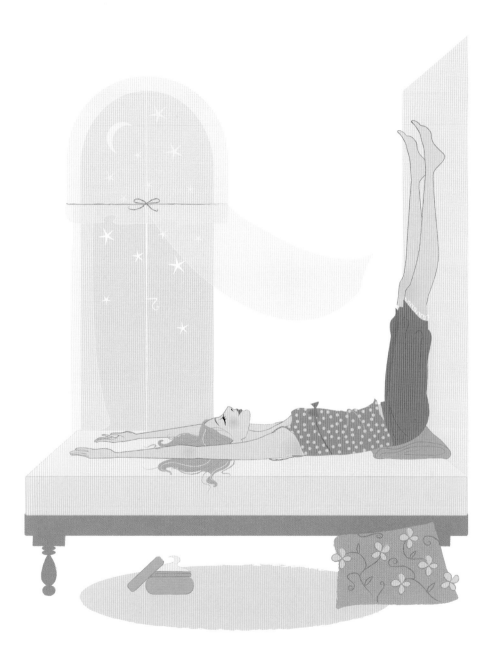

Wallflower

Viparita Karani variation – Simple Inverted variation

>>> How it works...

Roll up a blanket and place it against the wall. Lie down and place your buttocks on the blanket so that your legs are straight up against the wall. Stretch your arms out past your head. Inhale and exhale gently and deeply through your nose. Count to at least to six every time you inhale or exhale. The longer and more even your breaths, the more intense the calming effect. And while you're at it, dream a little.

<<< *The benefits*
Stimulates circulation in the torso and stomach area. Relaxes the nervous system. Calms. Combats headaches.

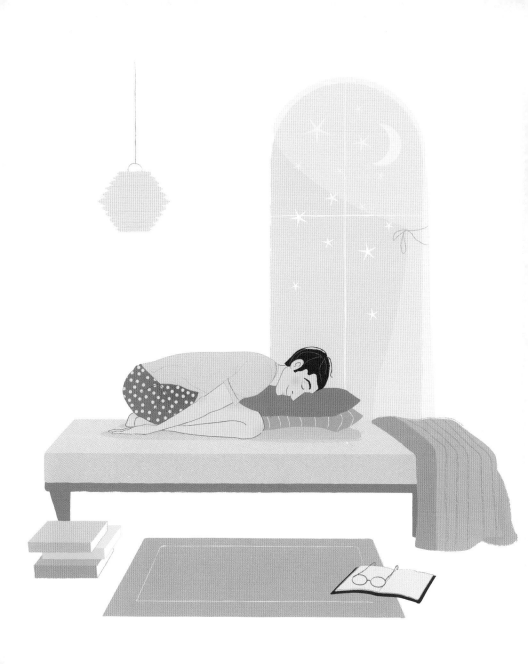

La-La-La

Salamba Balasana variation – Supported Child's variation

>>> How it works...

Kneel on the bed and sit on your heels. Spread your thighs wide enough to place a pile of towels between them. If you have knee problems, place a rolled up towel behind your knees, between your thighs and calves. Now, with your hands either behind you palms up or stretched out in front of you palms down, slowly lean your torso forwards. Inhale and exhale deeply through your nose. Each time you inhale or exhale, try to count to at least six. The higher you can count, the greater the calming effect you'll feel. Linger in the position for as long as it feels good – ideally, five to ten minutes.

<<< The benefits

Stretches the entire back. Relieves tension. Stretches the thigh muscles. Creates deep relaxation. Calms.

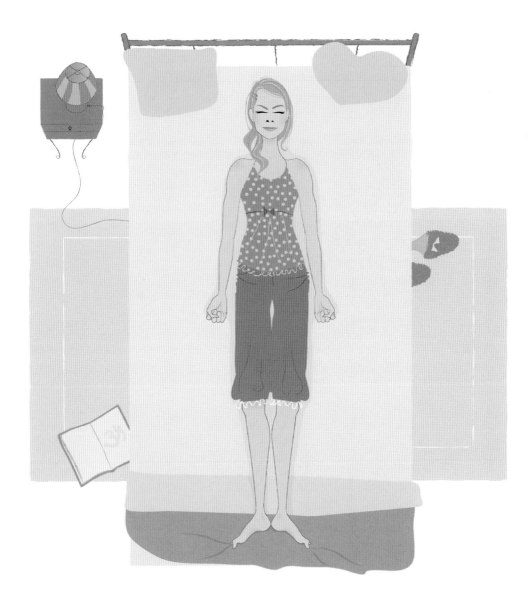

Squeezing Lemons

Shavasana variation – Corpse variation

>>> How it works...

Lie still on the bed. Keep your legs straight and together with your heels touching. Relax your toes and point them outwards. Keep your hands at your sides, palms up, slightly away from your body. Inhale and exhale slowly and deeply through your nose. Lie and breathe like this for five breaths. On the next inhale flex all the muscles in your body as hard as you can. Hold your breath when you do this and count to five. Then exhale and and release.

Repeat this exercise five times. Then remain in shavasana until you fall asleep. Sweet dreams.

<<< The benefits
Calms you down. Releases tension. Regenerates the mind and nervous system. Combats insomnia.

An Afterword and...

Excuse me, can you tell me the way to greater happiness, please?
Actually, we already have within ourselves everything we need in life:
love, longing and the awareness of ourselves and the things around us.
We only really need to learn again to trust completely our knowledge
and understanding.
I'm convinced that we are able to discover exactly what we really want out
of life. Simply take a minute to sit and write down four short-term and
long-term goals for yourself. From the time I began clearly setting my goals,
and then continued to adjust, compare and renew them four times a year
with each new season, my life has improved immensely. It is a fact that we
experience a feeling of contentment when we are able to manifest our
ideas, visions and goals. Often I feel as though I've handed my goals over
to a higher force and can completely let go of other less significant things.
Try it yourself. Take your list of goals and put it in a safe place. You'll be
astonished at how the positive energy will work for you

…Acknowledgements

I thank my wonderful family – my husband James, my children Christopher, Liam and, of course, Daniel –, my parents and my siblings Ralph and Sonja. I'm deeply grateful to Isabelle Follath for her wonderful illustrations; to Andrea Walter, without whom I could never have sorted out my thoughts; and to Greta Andreas, who quite simply organized everything. I thank Kim and Sören for their trust and for establishing the Yoga You Yoga Center in Palma; my yoga instructors; and everybody who has always believed in my dream. I thank my incredibly important friends and partners, Isabell, Maria, Doris, Astrid, Dana, Netti, Katja, Sandra, Kai, Julie, Angela, Patrizia, Carde, Sabrina, Nathalia and Andreas. I also thank Sönke, my all-round co-ordinator; my editor, Marion Schulz; and my proofreader, Rita Maria Güther, who stuck with me for each deadline. I thank the publishers, especially Georg Kessler and Ulrich Ehrlenspiel, for finding the right space for an atypical book. And I thank all the people who supported me so incredibly, but who I can't name here because I can use only 17 lines for acknowledgements.

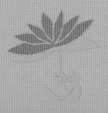

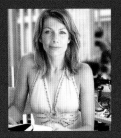

Ursula Karven is a mother of three and an actress who has appeared in many German and international TV and film productions over the past 20 years. She was born in Ulm, Germany, in 1964, and now lives with her family on Mallorca. From 1993 to 2005, she was based in California where she began to practice yoga. Her wish since then has been to share her experience of yoga with as many people as possible. After her best seller "Yoga für die Seele" ("Yoga for the Soul") and her children's book "Sina und die Yogakatze" ("Sina and the Yoga Cat"), "Yoga on the Go" shows us that we can use yoga exercises to transform everyday situations into meaningful experiences. Indeed, she developed the system as a way of juggling the challenges of family life, her company, her film work and her own yoga studio. The more pressure she's under, the more breaks she takes. So don't be astonished if you happen to see Ursula Karven standing upside-down in a plane, or on one leg in an elevator, or with her arms stretched out over her head at the supermarket.

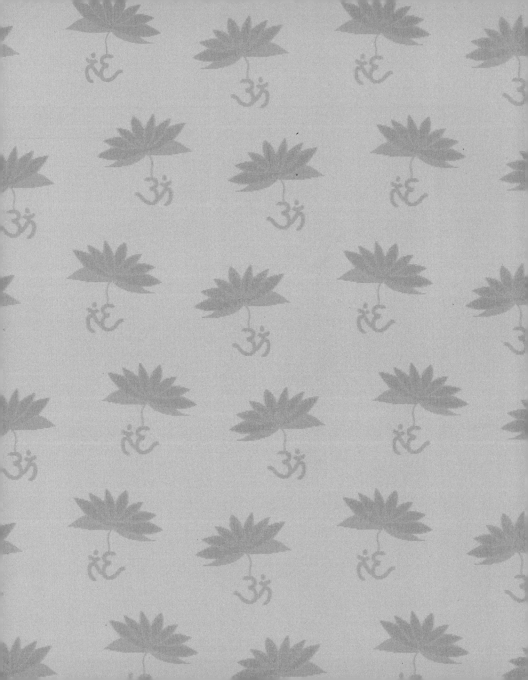